The Essential Guide to

Cervical Cancer

MARY LUNNEN

Published in Great Britain in 2018 by
need2know
Remus House
Coltsfoot Drive
Peterborough
PE2 9BF
Telephone 01733 898103
www.need2knowbooks.co.uk

Contents

Foreword

When I started working in the field of cervical cancer prevention in the mid-1980s, the cause of cervical cancer was still uncertain. There were many experts who did not believe that infection with the human papilloma virus (HPV) was important, and even more doctors who were quite unaware of any connection. It is almost unbelievable that, in such a short time, we have gone from debate about any possible role of HPV, to a vaccine which will prevent the infection and thus cervical cancer. Is it any wonder that, with the science moving so fast, many people, including doctors and nurses, have found it hard to keep up? With new information appearing all the time, often contradicting what came before, many people are confused and misinformed.

This book is written from the perspective of someone who has lived through the process of having an abnormal smear and undergoing treatment. As such, it offers invaluable insights into common concerns and gives practical advice on what to do and how to cope at every stage. It should help women and their families to understand the issues involved in both prevention and treatment of cervical cancer and thus empower them to make reasoned decisions.

Dr Anne Szarewski
Wolfson Institute of Preventive Medicine, London

Introduction

With the update of this book during 2018, I have the opportunity both to celebrate what has changed in the way of awareness and prevention of cervical cancer, and to urge women to be aware of symptoms. Women are still dying of this disease, which is potentially preventable.

I also have the opportunity to celebrate the positive reviews the initial publication received in 2010, for example, this extract from a longer review by Susan Quilliam (in the *Journal of Family Planning and Reproductive Health Care*, Volume 36, Number 3, July 2010 , pp. 174-174(1)).

I bought Susan's book *Positive Smear* many years ago when I was being treated and found the combination of expert knowledge and individual experiences extremely helpful.

"As someone who has had their own brush with CIN3, I am always on the lookout for good books aimed at those who want to inform and empower themselves around the issue of smear tests, positive smear results and cervical cancer. So, I am delighted at this new addition to a currently under-resourced field.

Three adjectives describe the book: compassionate, comprehensive, cancer-focused. Let's take these one by one."

There is not room to include the whole review here, you can find the full text on my website. (daretoblossom.co.uk) After much praise for the book, Susan expressed her concern that women who have not been diagnosed with cervical cancer should not miss out on the useful information, ending her review with these words:

"In short, I love this book. But I do hope that the fullest possible target market will not be misdirected by its cancer-focused title, and so fail to benefit from its superbly comprehensive and compassionate approach."

I hope that you will find this book useful and informative for all aspects of your gynaecological heath.

Mary Lunnen June 2018.

Acknowledgements

Thank you to everyone who has helped in any way with this book. In particular, my two medical experts, Mary White, of PDI International Ltd, and the person Mary introduced me to, Dr Alison St John, consultant pathologist at the Royal Cornwall Hospital. Mary and Alison have been wonderfully generous with their time and expert advice.

I am honoured and delighted that the renowned and respected expert in this field, Dr Anne Szarewski, has taken time from her hectic schedule to write the forword to this book. Her writing was a great support to me personally during my own treatment, and also during my work on this title.

My thanks also to Amy Brownlie, Emma Gubb and Alison Cross of Need2Know who have been patient and expert in their guidance of my work on this book.

Disclaimer

This book is only for general information about cervical cancer and is not intended to replace medical advice. You should consult your GP or healthcare practitioner for individual medical advice about treatment of cervical cancer or any worries or concerns you may have. The factual material in this book is drawn from a variety of sources, which are listed in the help list and book list. All facts and figures are as up-to-date as possible, but please refer to these sources for the most recent research.

1

What is Cervical Cancer?

nformation is the greatest aid in dealing with health issues. 'Cancer' is a word with so many frightening associations that it provokes an immediate reaction, and when it is combined with what may be an embarrassing area of the body it may feel even harder to ask questions.

This chapter will give you all the basic facts about cervical cancer so you can be well prepared for anything you need to deal with, whether prevention or treatment. Later chapters in the book will give you more detailed information. You can choose to jump straight to these or read the book from the beginning.

The help list at the end of the book gives details of where to access more help and support. For overview information, the NHS Choices website (see help list) is an excellent starting point, and I am grateful for their permission to quote from the material. Simply follow the links, via the A-Z, to 'C' for cancer, and then to 'cervical cancer'. One resource you will find is a video by Andy Nordin, a gynaecological oncologist, who explains cervical cancer in a friendly and understandable way.

The cervix

To start with some background facts, the cervix is part of a woman's reproductive organs. It is the lower part of the womb (also called the uterus), and is a passageway connecting the womb and the vagina. The cervix is sometimes called the neck of the womb.

The functions of the cervix

When a girl starts her period, the cervix allows the menstrual blood to flow out of the womb and leave the body. During sex, the cervix allows the man's sperm to enter the womb, and if the sperm fertilises an egg then pregnancy can occur. When a woman gives birth, the cervical canal widens (dilates) to allow the baby to be born.

During cervical screening (also known as the smear test), the nurse takes a sample of cells from the cervix to check for any changes. You will find more information about screening in chapter 3.

Cancer

Cancer is caused when the normal replacement process of cells in the body gets out of control and produces a tumour. You can have a tumour without having cancer. This is known as a benign tumour and the cells do not spread to other parts of the body. Benign tumours can sometimes cause a problem if they grow large and press on surrounding tissues, for example in the brain.

A malignant tumour is one where the cells tend to spread into other areas of the body, via the blood or the lymph glands, and this is what is known as a cancerous tumour. There are many different types of cancer which are identified by what is called the primary site, so for example, as well as cervical cancer, there is breast cancer, lung cancer, bone cancer and many others.

Secondary cancer

If the cancer cells do spread, other tumours may develop at different places in the body. This is known as a secondary cancer or metastasis. There is more information about this in chapter 7.

Causes of cervical cancer

The precise reason why one cell should start dividing out of control and become a cancer cell is unknown. Research is going on all around the world into the causes of all types of cancer and a number of risk factors for cervical cancer have been established.

They are known as risk factors because they are associated with the development of cervical cancer. This does not necessarily mean they cause the cancer, nor does it mean that if you have cancer you will have all or any of these factors in your life.

Risk factors

HPV

This is associated with 99.7% of cases of cervical cancer. HPVs are a group of more than 100 viruses. Some of these cause genital warts, common warts and verrucas.

Other types of HPV cause changes in the cells of the cervix which are known as cervical intra-epithelial neoplasia (CIN), and it is this that is detected by cervical screening tests. These changes are known as pre-cancerous. CIN can develop into cancer if left untreated, but in some cases the cells will return to normal by themselves.

The doctor will advise on the best course of action for each patient based on individual circumstances, which are of course different for everyone. See chapter 3 on the screening programme for more information. Most people who have HPV do not develop CIN or cancer; the infection simply increases the risk.

HPVs are nearly always passed on by sexual contact and this can make it a sensitive and upsetting subject for girls and women, and for their families. It means that the risk of becoming infected with HPV increases if you begin having sex at a young age, and goes up with the number of sexual partners you have. This is the reason why vaccines effective against HPVs have been developed and why the vaccination programme put into place in the UK (and elsewhere in the world) is aimed at young girls before they become sexually active. See more detailed information in chapter 2.

Even if you have been vaccinated, it is still important not to have unprotected intercourse; you must use a condom as the vaccine does not protect against all types of HPV, or against other sorts of sexually transmitted infections (STIs).

However, it is not true that if you are diagnosed with HPV infection, CIN or cervical cancer, that you have had many sexual partners. It is also not true that you will definitely develop one of these conditions if you were young when you began having sex or if you have had a number of partners. Please see chapter 6 for more on helping you and your family deal with the emotions and feelings raised by coping with all these issues.

Smoking

Research has shown that there is a link between smoking and the risk of developing a number of different cancers, including cervical cancer. It is not known precisely why this is; it is thought to be due to chemicals from the smoke entering the blood and being carried to cells around the body.

Having children young or several children

Again, research shows that women who have their first baby before 17 have double the risk of developing cervical cancer compared with women whose first child is born when they are over 25. This could be associated with the fact that these people became sexually active at quite a young age. Also women with three or more children have an increased risk, although it is not yet clear why this should be the case.

Taking the pill

Using the contraceptive pill for more than 10 years may slightly increase the risk of developing cervical cancer. However, there are many health benefits associated with taking the pill and you should discuss your personal situation with your GP. For general information, see *The Pill – An Essential Guide* (Need2Know).

Low immune system

If your immune system is weakened for any reason, you may be less resistant to any illness. The immune system helps to destroy abnormal cells such as cancer cells as well as protect the body against infections such as HPV.

Factors that weaken your immune system include HPV and smoking (which have already been mentioned), HIV or AIDS, or by drugs taken to suppress the body's immune system after an organ transplant to reduce the chance of rejection.

The debate over stress

Many people believe that stress can cause cancer; however, research studies have been carried out without producing any conclusive evidence of this. It could be that stress can weaken the immune system and make you generally more susceptible to the effects of the other factors described above, but again there is no scientific proof of this at present.

Please remember that these are risk factors only – none of them will mean that you will get cancer. All risk is relative and none of us can remove all risk from our lives.

The most important thing you can do to help yourself, or your daughter, is to follow a healthy lifestyle now, including taking advantage of the HPV vaccination programme if that is right for you, and to attend cervical screenings when invited by your GP.

Types of cancer of the cervix

There are various types of cervical cancer, the most common one accounting for 80% of all cases in the UK.

Squamous cell carcinoma

The most common type of cervical cancer is called squamous cell carcinoma (or cancer). The squamous cells are the flat cells that cover the surface of the cervix, and squamous cell cancers are diagnosed in approximately 80% of all cervical cancers.

Adenocarcinoma

Adenocarcinoma develops from the glandular cells that line the cervical canal (endocervix). Adenocarcinoma starts in the cervical canal and can therefore be more difficult to detect using cervical screening tests. This type of cervical cancer makes up approximately 20% of cases.

Rare types of cervical cancer

Other rare types of cervical cancer include clear cell, adenosquamous cancers, small cell undifferentiated, lymphomas and sarcomas. These are extremely rare – so rare that they do not show up in the percentages given above. If you are concerned about these, or any other issues, the phone line staffed by cancer support specialists at Macmillan Cancer Support can give you more information (see help list).

Symptoms of cervical cancer

As I found myself, the symptoms of cervical cancer are not always obvious. There may not be any signs at all until it has reached an advanced stage. This is why it is extremely important for you to have regular cervical smear tests.

If cervical cancer does cause symptoms, the most common is abnormal bleeding, such as between periods or after sexual intercourse. In post-menopausal women (those who have stopped having periods), there may be new bleeding. Other symptoms of cervical cancer may include a smelly vaginal discharge and discomfort when having sex.

There are other conditions that have similar symptoms, so it is important that you visit your GP or practice nurse if you have any of the symptoms talked about here. It can be embarrassing to talk about, so it might help to make a list of questions or points you want to mention.

'As I found myself, the symptoms of cervical cancer are not always obvious.'

You may be able to ask to see a female GP, and be assured that all GPs are trained to help people with worries such as these. When I had my first (and only) abnormal cervical screening test, I had already been experiencing bleeding after intercourse but did not realise that it was significant.

In hindsight, I cannot believe that for some reason I did not ask my GP about it – I would encourage anyone who experiences any symptoms to get help immediately. I hope this book will raise awareness of the signs to look out for and enable you to act more quickly than I did.

Diagnosis of cervical cancer

Cervical screening is a test to look for abnormal changes in the cells of the cervix. Some cell changes may, if left untreated, go on to develop into cancer. It is not a test to diagnose cervical cancer itself, so if your cervical screening test shows any indication of abnormal cells, your GP will refer you for a follow-up. This may be taking another cervical screening test sample, or other tests or investigations as described below.

Abnormal cells often return to normal by themselves. If this does not happen, or if the doctor decides it is best for you not to wait, they may be treated before they ever have a chance to become cancer cells.

Early diagnosis of cervical cancer is essential for successful treatment of the condition. Your GP will arrange any tests that are necessary and will refer you to a specialist who can give you gynaecological treatment and advice.

Further tests are needed to make a diagnosis, and these may include:

- Colposcopy – this usually takes place as an outpatient at your local hospital and is an examination using a small light and microscope. Sometimes a biopsy (sample) is taken at the same time and you may have a local anaesthetic to ensure that no pain is felt.

- A cone biopsy where a larger tissue sample is taken. This may remove the abnormal area if it is small (microinvasive), or be used for diagnosis.

- A physical examination under anaesthetic, during which a biopsy of the womb lining is often taken.

If cervical cancer is diagnosed, further tests will be conducted, and may include one or more of these:

- Blood tests.

- X-ray.

- Ultrasound of the pelvic area.

- Computerised tomography scan (CT scan).

- Magnetic resonance imaging (MRI scan).

'Abnormal bleeding is the most common symptom, particularly after intercourse – an indication to see your doctor.'

Andy Nordin, NHS Choices.

Summing Up

Just hearing the word cancer can be frightening and sometimes people react by trying to ignore or forget all about it. However, in recent years big advances have been made in detection and treatment of this disease.

You can help yourself, your daughter, family, students or friends by being well informed on the symptoms, being aware of the importance of attending cervical screening appointments and talking to your GP if you are at all concerned.

2

Prevention

For all of us, the ideal is to prevent any illness occurring. So to help prevent cervical cancer, there are a number of ways in which we can minimise the risks posed by the factors that we just discussed.

Safe sex

As mentioned earlier, one of the known causes of cervical cancer is infection with certain types of HPV. This is transmitted by sexual activity and the risk of contracting it increases with the number of partners you have. Research also indicates that the risk is increased for a woman if her partner has had many previous relationships (see *Preventing Cervical Cancer* by Dr Anne Szarewski).

There is more discussion about this below in the section on vaccination. One of the concerns about the vaccination programme is that some people think it may encourage girls to think it's safe to have sex. The whole subject is a sensitive one and everyone, including parents and young people, will benefit from obtaining expert advice.

Protection against other diseases

It is important to realise that the vaccines do not protect against anything other than the two strains of HPV known as HPV 16 and 18. To protect against other STIs such as chlamydia, syphilis or HIV (and other strains of HPV), it is necessary to use a condom. For more information on looking after your sexual health, see *Sexually Transmitted Infections – The Essential Guide* (Need2Know).

Contraception

No method of contraception is 100% effective, and many people choose to use another method such as the pill or the cap. To gain maximum protection against both STIs and unwanted pregnancy, it is advised to use more than one type of contraception.

Get expert advice

The easiest way to decide what is best for you as an individual is to see your GP or visit a family planning clinic. Many areas have drop-in clinics and centres aimed at teenagers to help them feel less embarrassed about the whole subject. You can also talk to health advisors or doctors at the local hospital genito-urinary (GUM) clinic. They are experts in sexual health and the consultation is done in complete confidence with no feedback to your GP.

If you're reading this as a teenager, or parent of a teenager, you'll be interested to know that one reliable source is the Teens First for Health website (see help list). Here you'll have all your questions answered in a straightforward and friendly style.

Vaccination

So, what is the vaccination programme, who can benefit, and are there any risks?

Vaccines

Two vaccines have been licensed for use in the UK. These are Cervarix®, manufactured by GlaxoSmithKline, and Gardasil®, developed by Sanofi Pasteur MSD. Both vaccines protect against the two most common types of HPV (known as types 16 and 18), that cause cervical cancer.

Cervarix® has been chosen for use in the UK and the vaccination programme started in 2008, with different timings in England, Scotland, Wales and Northern Ireland. The NHS Immunisation website (see help list), states that the reason for the choice was that the company scored higher against pre-agreed criteria. If you are interested to know more about this process you can find detailed information by visiting the website.

The programme

In England girls in the age ranges 12-13 years and 17-18 years have been offered vaccinations since September 2008, with a 'catch-up' programme aiming to make sure that all girls born since 1 September 1990 will have been covered by the end of the 2009/2010 academic year.

Where the vaccinations take place varies. Younger girls are more likely to receive theirs in school, with older girls seeing their GP. Three doses are given over a six month period.

Similar programmes are running in Scotland, Northern Ireland and Wales. The help list gives details of the websites containing information. There is, at the time of writing, no vaccination programme in the Republic of Ireland, though some GPs may provide the service for a fee.

Are there any side effects?

Almost all medicines have some side effects that are discovered when they are tested before being approved. In the case of the HPV vaccines some of the side effects that might be experienced are listed on the Teens First for Health website (see help list) in the 'Ask the Doc' section, as:

- Headache.
- Aching muscles.
- Redness and soreness around the site of the injection.
- Fever.
- Feeling and being sick.
- Stomach pain.
- Diarrhoea.
- Itching and/or a rash.
- Dizziness.

'Almost all medicines have some side effects that are discovered when they are tested before being approved.'

You or your daughter will be given information about possible side effects when the vaccination is done and you should contact your GP if you experience any of these. In nearly all cases these effects are very mild, if felt at all, and are rarely a reason to stop having the vaccinations.

On rare occasions some girls have experienced more serious side effects such as an allergic reaction or anaphylactic shock that causes breathing difficulties. The medical staff who give the vaccinations are trained to deal with any emergencies such as this that may arise.

There is also research evidence to show that some reported side effects can be coincidental and would have occurred anyway (i.e. the vaccination did not cause them, see CA Siegrist, 2007).

Should I (or my daughter) have the vaccination?

'The HPV vaccination programme is recommended as part of efforts to prevent cervical cancer developing.'

If you are being offered the vaccination it is important to examine the facts for yourself and take advice from reliable sources of information. Every parent has to make their own decision with their daughter on what is right for them.

The HPV vaccination programme is recommended as part of efforts to prevent cervical cancer developing. If girls and young women can avoid contracting HPVs, this can be an effective way to reduce the risk of pre-cancerous changes occurring in the cells of the cervix, and perhaps developing cancer.

There has been controversy about the vaccination programme in the media and some concerns that it could be encouraging young girls to become sexually active. The vaccination has to be given before this occurs as it prevents infection but does not eliminate a HPV once you have developed it. Therefore the ideal time is when a girl is young.

A well-known researcher and writer, Dr Anne Szarewski, has been working in this field for many years. She and her colleagues are convinced of the value of the vaccination programme and recommend that if possible it be extended to older women, and also that it is linked to individual records of cervical screening. (If you are interested in reading about these views they are contained in a paper describing a 'round-table' discussion on the subject, see A Szarweski et al., 2009 and the book list for details of Dr Szarewski's books.)

You should also be aware that even if you are exposed to HPV it does not mean that you will develop cervical cancer. It is still not known for sure why some women develop the disease and others do not. All you can do is take sensible steps to do your best to reduce the risks.

Finding reliable information on the Internet

The Internet is a great source of information, but it also contains much that is inaccurate and even completely wrong, so it needs to be treated with caution. The help list at the end of this book contains recommendations for sources of good information.

As already mentioned, the Teens First for Health website has an excellent section which discusses the pros and cons of the vaccination (see help list). Whether you're a teenager or a parent, you'll find straightforward information on safe sex, cervical screening and many other topics.

How can I help myself?

For our own good health in general, it is important to develop awareness of our bodies and how we feel. As women, especially if we have children and maybe elderly family to care for as well, we tend to look after everybody else before ourselves.

Balance in life

As well as being a writer, I work as a life coach, and a large part of that work is giving people (female or male) the time and space to put their own needs first for once. There is more about a healthy lifestyle below, and ideally this is not something we just think about occasionally. Making a habit of looking regularly at the balance of our lives can be one way of making sure we do everything we can to help ourselves stay fit and well.

I feel it is not simply what people call 'work/life balance', though that is important of course. It is about balance between all parts of your life: family, friends, hobbies, work, exercise, sport, relaxation, creativity, spirituality or religion and learning – whatever is important to you.

Using a wheel of life exercise

One of the first exercises many coaches offer their clients is some variation on the wheel of life exercise. Here is one version for you to try which will show you very graphically if your life is out of balance in any area.

The wheel of life exercise allows you to determine whether you are focusing too much on one part of your life and so neglecting other parts. You can draw your own wheel on a piece of paper and you can change the headings as you wish, or add more.

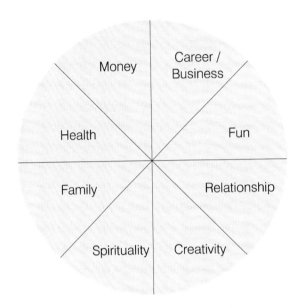

Regarding the centre of the wheel as zero and the outer edge as 10, rank your level of satisfaction with each life area by drawing a curved line to create a new outer edge. The new perimeter of the circle represents the wheel of life. How bumpy would the ride be if this were a real wheel?

Your wheel shows you the degree to which you are satisfied with your level of balance in your life. Which are your low spots – the areas you are least satisfied with? Can you develop some easy steps to rebalance these areas? (You can read more about this approach in my book, *Dare to Blossom: Coaching and Creativity*.)

I have found it useful to repeat this exercise at regular intervals as it gives me an opportunity to regularly 'check in with myself' on how I am feeling at any time. The balance naturally shifts and changes all the time as we turn our focus to different parts of our lives.

For me, the beauty of using this visual approach is that it also emphasises how each part of the wheel is inter-linked and affects the other parts. For example, if I am worried about the security of my job, it can have an effect on my health. Conversely, if I am unwell it may mean that I am less able to do my job well.

This is just one suggestion for how you can help yourself to feel more in control of your life and your health.

What can I do for my daughter?

If you are the parent of a daughter, you naturally want to do the best for her. Reading the following sections, perhaps together, will enable you to support her to live a healthy lifestyle.

What if my daughter won't talk to me?

Depending on the age of your daughter, the ideal is to have a good relationship where she feels comfortable talking to you about these sensitive subjects. We all know that relationships are not always ideal, especially in those rocky teenage years, so if communication between you is difficult, is there someone else she can get support from? It may be an aunt or grandmother, an older family friend, a teacher, youth worker, nurse or GP.

Healthy lifestyle

Earlier, I suggested ways that you could look at whether you have a healthy and happy balance in life. You may have decided to draw up your own wheel of life. If you did, what did it show you? You may have decided you would like to lose weight or eat a more healthy diet, or take up a new sport or pastime to encourage you to get out in the fresh air. All these things will help you become as fit and well as possible and make it less likely that you will develop any illness.

Will living a healthy lifestyle stop cancer?

The short answer is no. Living a healthy lifestyle will help you avoid many problems and perhaps reduce the risk of developing cancer. Avoiding the proven risk factors such as smoking and unsafe sex is highly advisable for all sorts of reasons.

However, it is also important to realise that you should not blame yourself if you do develop cancer. Dr Alison St John, consultant pathologist, emphasised in a personal communication to me:

'Living a healthy lifestyle will help you avoid many problems and perhaps reduce the risk of developing cancer. Avoiding the proven risk factors such as smoking and unsafe sex is highly advisable for all sorts of reasons.'

'It is not fair to suggest that healthy living is a strong factor in preventing cancer. I say that because of the number of women I have encountered who have lived "healthy" lives and who are devastated that despite their efforts, which they thought were protective, they have developed cancer. Obesity is certainly a factor in endometrial, ovarian and breast cancers but not in cervical cancer. Smoking is an important factor. I do realise though that it is important that women learn to listen to their bodies, and I think it is very helpful to suggest to young teenagers that they take responsibility for their wellbeing.'

What is a 'healthy lifestyle'?

'Smoking not only causes lung cancer but also increases the risk of you developing other cancers, including cervical cancer.'

Good question! There is so much about this subject in the media and often those reports can seem to contradict each other. For example, one may say we should not eat butter at all, then another that moderate amounts can be good for us.

A healthy lifestyle can include diet, exercise and not smoking, plus relaxation and time for hobbies, friends and family. There are many books and information sources about all of these topics, so the next sections will very briefly look at diet, smoking and exercise.

Diet

A balanced diet will include fresh fruit and vegetables, protein (such as meat, fish, eggs or cheese) and carbohydrates (e.g. bread, potatoes, rice, pasta or beans). Sometimes people decide to take supplements of vitamins or minerals, but if you are generally healthy and eating a balanced diet you probably would not need these.

As always, if in doubt always get expert advice. There is good information on the Teens First for Health website, under 'healthy eating' and on NHS Choices in the 'live well' section. This is a huge subject and, as with many health issues, not all the experts agree, so it is up to you to get the best advice and decide what works for you. For more information on healthy eating, see *Student Cookbook – Healthy Eating* (Need2Know).

Smoking

As mentioned in chapter 1, it is proven that smoking not only causes lung cancer but also increases the risk of you developing other cancers, including cervical cancer. Smoking also increases the risk of other serious problems such as heart disease and strokes.

There are free services available via the NHS to help you give up smoking, so do take advantage of these if you feel that you are unable to achieve this on your own. A good place to start is the NHS Choices website (see help list), where you will find ideas to keep yourself motivated and links to local services.

Exercise

An important part of a healthy lifestyle is exercise. Find something you enjoy doing that won't become just something else on your 'should' list, and make it a new regular habit.

If you enjoy activities with friends, get them involved too. Many people get enormous satisfaction out of taking on challenges for charity such as the Race for Life organised by Cancer Research UK at venues all around the country. Maybe, you prefer quiet walks in the countryside or classes such as yoga or pilates.

Cervical screening

Chapter 3 covers the topic of the cervical screening programme in detail. It is mentioned here to emphasise that it is part of prevention of cervical cancer.

If going for regular cervical screening checks is seen as something to be afraid of, it makes it hard. Thinking of it as part of the whole programme that you are putting into place for yourself can help you see it as another positive step you are taking to look after your body.

Chapter 3 will explain the whole process in detail and help you to see it as an early warning system that can enable you to make sure that any potential problems are investigated and treated long before they develop into something serious. You may be referred to the colposcopy clinic at your local hospital for further investigation or for treatment; this is also covered briefly in chapter 3 and in more detail in chapter 4.

Summing Up

'Prevention is better than cure' is an old saying, and none the less true for that.

This chapter has summarised some of the things you can do for yourself and encourage your family and friends to do, which will reduce the chance of developing a serious illness like cervical cancer.

Taking responsibility for doing what you can to stay healthy can become a positive habit and many types of exercise can be enjoyed in the company of others or by yourself, whichever suits you best.

However, as emphasised earlier, cancer is a complex disease and all the causes are not yet known. So, in spite of all your best efforts, you may still find yourself being offered treatment for abnormal cells or for cervical cancer. You will find more information in the chapters that follow to explain what might be offered to you.

The Screening Programme

As promised, this chapter will give a basic outline of what the cervical cancer screening programme involves. The book list contains references to other reading that will take you into more detail if you wish. The most up-to-date information can be found on the NHS cancer screening website for the programme (see help list).

Statistics

Cervical Screening Programme in England 2016-2017

The Cancer Research UK website is also a useful source of statistical information.

For example, the following figures are drawn from their summary statistics:

- At 31 March 2017, the percentage of eligible women (aged 25 to 64) who were recorded as screened adequately within the specified period was 72.0 per cent. This compares with 72.7 per cent at 31 March 2016 and 75.4 per cent at 31 March 2012.

- A total of 4.45 million women aged 25 to 64 were invited for screening in 2016-17, representing an increase of 5.6 per cent from 2015-16 when 4.21 million women were invited.

- In total, 3.18 million women aged 25 to 64 years were tested in 2016-17, an increase of 2.9 per cent from 2015-16 when 3.09 million women were tested.

- Of samples submitted by GPs and NHS Community Clinics, 94.8 per cent of test results were returned Negative.

Ref: "Cervical Screening Programme, England – 2016 -2017, pub November 07, 2017.

Table 1.1: Cervical Screening Programme Results, UK by country, target age group and target frequency

	Target age group	Frequency of invites
England	25-64	Every 3 or 5 years
Wales	20-64	Every 3 years
Scotland	20-60	Normal practice, every 3 years
Northern Ireland	20-64	Every 3 or 5 years

The target age group and frequency of invite for each country of the UK. (Source: www.cancerresearchuk.org, accessed 1 December 2009.)

A note on statistics

Statistics always show the figures for large groups of people (known as 'populations') and not what may happen to you as an individual.

An excellent and clear explanation of statistics can be found on the Cancer Help website under 'about statistics' (see help list).

For example, in connection with the point above, the Cancer Help website explains:

'If 65% of people with your type of cancer responded to a treatment, then there is a two out of three chance that you will too. But no one can say definitely whether your cancer will respond to that treatment.'

Statistics can give you general information about types of cancer and the effectiveness of various treatments, but the final decision should be based on consultations with your doctors about your individual situation.

What is screening?

It cannot be emphasised too often that the cervical screening programme does not look for cancer. The sample of cells taken is examined under a microscope to look for signs of abnormal cells. It is not a test with a definite answer like the one you would expect if a biopsy (a small piece of body tissue) was sent to the laboratory for analysis.

A good example of screening is what happens to your hand luggage at airport security. Your bag is put into a machine and the screener looks at the image of bag contents. The screener can usually detect something that shouldn't be there, such as a pair of scissors. Screening is not as accurate as opening the bag and checking through all the things in it one by one – that would take too long to be practical. In cervical screening, the slide with your cells on it is like the piece of baggage being screened.

Dr Alison St John explains that most abnormalities are detected but since each individual cell cannot be scrutinised on its own, occasional abnormalities may be overlooked. This is one reason for attending screening regularly; if abnormalities persist, they have a good chance of being picked up – if not the first time, then the second or third time.

'It cannot be emphasised too often that the cervical screening programme does not look for cancer. The sample of cells that is taken is examined under a microscope to look for signs of abnormal cells.'

What happens in the surgery?

When you go to the surgery for your first cervical screening appointment (or at any time for that matter), you may be nervous, or you may see it as a nuisance.

If you are nervous, ask to have a talk to the nurse before your appointment, or look at some of the information sources given in the help list. Your GP or practice nurse will take the sample (also known as a 'smear' because in the past the cells collected from your cervix were 'smeared' onto the slide).

You will be asked to remove your pants and lie on your back with your legs apart so that the nurse can take the sample. A piece of medical equipment known as a speculum is used. It is placed in your vagina and then opened so that the nurse can insert a small brush that collects the sample cells.

The test itself involves taking a sample of cells from the cervix which is put onto a glass slide and sent to a laboratory to be checked for abnormal cells. In the past staff known as cytologists would then view each slide under a microscope. However, the development of liquid based cytology (LBC) has improved the accuracy of the tests by making any abnormal cells more easily detectable by the cytologists. As a result, in this process the sample takers now transfer the material into a pot of liquid, and this liquid is then transferred onto a slide in the laboratory. (More detail on this process is provided later in the chapter.)

Why is it important?

This test is important because if abnormal cells are detected early, they can be monitored or treated which helps prevent them ever developing into cervical cancer cells. So, if your GP invites you to a screening appointment, make sure you go!

My own experience was that I had been attending every three years and had never had an abnormal result to my tests. Then in 1994, I did have one. This was followed up by a referral to the colposcopy clinic (see chapter 4), and then to further treatment which prevented me developing more advanced cancer and probably saved my life. So, I am eternally grateful that there is a system such as this.

When I have my test, how will I know that it will be done correctly?

The NHS cancer screening programme (NHSCSP) is a national body that is responsible for cancer screening. This includes close monitoring of all the services concerning cancer screening, including the training of nurses and GPs. It also sets the standards for the training of taking smears.

Mary White, who runs training courses for the nurses working on the cervical cancer screening programme in Devon and Cornwall for Professional Development International, kindly answered the following questions for me.

Q. What kind of training do cervical screening nurses have?

A. All health professionals who take smears must be registered. This means doctors, GPs, and nurses who are named on a professional register. So it does not include health care assistants and advanced practitioners. This is because it is important to have the professional knowledge to support the taking of a smear. Many of the smears are taken by nurses, especially in general practice surgeries. All smear takers must complete a basic course with two assessments and monitoring over the following six or nine months.

You may occasionally have a student in training when you have your smear taken, but you can be reassured that they will be supervised and assessed by an experienced, approved smear taker. Only when the assessor is satisfied that the results are of the correct standard can the smear taker take them unsupervised. When the smear taker has achieved sufficient number and standard of results they will be certified as competent.

Q. What happens after the initial training?

A. All smear takers should attend an update every three years. This training is normally organised by the local clinical commissioning group (CCG) who are responsible for reporting back to the regional and national bodies of the NHSCSP. As well as the three yearly training updates, smear takers must keep a check on their test results and make sure they are of the highest standard.

What happens to your specimen when it reaches the laboratory?

Dr Alison St John, consultant pathologist at Royal Cornwall Hospital, has kindly answered the following questions.

Q. What is the technical process when a sample is being checked?

The cells that are brushed from your cervix are put into pot of fluid. When this reaches the laboratory, the pot is put into a machine which extracts some of the cells and puts them on a glass slide. The cells are then stained with special dyes making them easy to see and recognise.

Q. What is the screening process?

The slide with the cells from your cervix is looked at through a microscope by a screener (a cytologist), a person trained to look at cervical smears and to recognise abnormalities. As there are about 50,000 cells on the slide, it would take too long to look carefully at each one individually. Instead, the screener moves the slide back and forwards on the microscope looking at all the cells.

If the screener detects an abnormality, he or she stops to look at the abnormal cell more carefully and marks its place on the slide with a felt tip marker. If the screener thinks there are no abnormal cells present, the slide is screened again by another screener, just as a precaution.

However, if the screener thinks there are abnormal cells present, the slide is passed to a more experienced person to look at. If he or she thinks there are abnormal cells present, the slide is then passed on to a doctor for his or her opinion.

The doctor makes the final decision and decides whether the woman should have her smear repeated at the usual time, repeated early, or if she should attend a colposcopy clinic where the cervix can be looked at by an expert. You can see that a lot of people look at the slides of cells from the cervix, so you can be confident that your smear is looked at thoroughly.

What is an abnormal smear?

Abnormal simply means that some cells in the sample look slightly different to normal healthy cells. If you get such a result, it could be possible that you've had what is called an inadequate sample taken. This means that either there were not enough cells present to make a judgement or they were obscured by blood or mucus.

Very rarely an inadequate sample may be due to a clerical error. Under pressure in a busy clinic, it may be that the smear taker omits to put vital information on the sample pot such as your date of birth. To ensure that every effort is made to avoid mistakes, the laboratory will refuse to process the sample unless the correct information is included.

When I had the test that led to my diagnosis, the nurse warned me that I might be recalled for another test as 'there is a bit of blood there'. The fact that she warned me of this was very helpful because when I did receive the news from my GP that my test result showed some abnormality, I was not overly worried. I was reassured that the hospital had decided to follow it up by an investigation at the colposcopy clinic.

Your smear result may be graded as showing mild, moderate or severe dyskaryosis. The word 'dyskaryosis' comes from the Greek words meaning 'abnormal nucleus', and the graded descriptions are what can be seen by the cytologist through the microscope. These changes are not cancer – they are changes to the cells that might possibly become cancer.

As described earlier, abnormal cells often disappear again without any treatment, so you may be asked to return for another test, either straightaway or more quickly than usual, perhaps in six or 12 months.

Does it mean I have cancer?

Many people become very worried when they receive a positive smear result, but it does not mean that you have cancer. It simply means that you have some cells that appear to be abnormal.

'Abnormal cells often disappear again without any treatment, so you may be asked to return for another test, either straight away or more quickly than usual, perhaps in six or 12 months.'

'A positive smear result does not mean that you have cancer.'

Your GP will explain what your results show and discuss with you the recommended course of action. In many cases, the best option is to wait and see if the next screening test reverts to normal as very often your body will deal with the abnormal cells itself. Also there is the possibility of a 'false positive' result, meaning that the cytologist viewing your sample slide thought there were abnormal cells present when there were actually none.

It is also possible to have a 'false negative' result, where there are abnormal cells but they are not picked up on the sample or not seen by the cytologist. This is why it is so important to keep to the regular appointments for your tests; if something is missed, it is unlikely to develop into something more serious in three years as the changes from 'abnormal' to 'cancer' cells are normally very slow. However, if you miss a test and there is a gap of six years, there is more of a risk of abnormal cells developing.

If necessary, your GP may refer you for further investigation to the colposcopy clinic at your local hospital (see chapter 4).

Summing Up

The cervical screening programme is the key part of the actions being taken to prevent women developing cervical cancer. The statistics below show that of all the millions of tests taken each year only a small number of women go on to develop cervical cancer. Cancer Research UK state on their website that:

- There are around 3,200 new cervical cancer cases in the UK every year, that's nearly 9 every day (2013-2015).

- Of these around 890 die each year.

It is vital that you do attend when you are invited even if you feel well and are busy with 'normal' life. Most of the women who die from cervical cancer have either never had a cervical screening test or did not attend their regular appointments.

If you are worried or nervous, please talk to your practice nurse or GP and use the organisations listed in the help list.

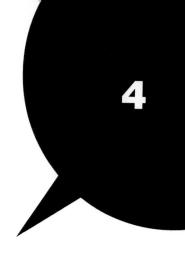

4

Treatment Following an Abnormal Result

This chapter gives an overview of all the possible treatments that you might be offered following the report of abnormal cells on your cervical screening test sample. The information will also be of use for anyone wanting further advice in this area.

The treatment for cervical cancer will be described in more detail in chapter 5.

Colposcopy investigations and treatments

Colposcopy is a difficult word to say, and that in itself can be a barrier to understanding what it is all about and being able to ask questions. There is a brief explanation here and the references and links provided will give you more information.

What is a colposcopy?

A colposcope is a device that allows the doctor to look more closely at your cervix using a large magnifying glass with a light attached. When you go into the room at the clinic, you will see a large machine that may look a little scary. However, the machine itself does not touch you or go inside your body; it is simply used to shine a light and enable the doctor to see a magnified view to check what has been found through the screening process.

Sometimes the colposcope is connected to video equipment and a screen so the pictures can be seen more easily by the doctor. You may be asked if you would like to watch the pictures too, but you can of course say no if you would rather not see them.

Before the examination

'You might like to prepare a list of questions to ask in advance as it is so easy to forget or not feel able to ask when you are there.'

The doctor will probably ask you when you had your last period, so it is useful to have that information written down to bring with you. If when you receive notification of your appointment it is at a time when you expect to be having your period, contact the clinic and ask for a change of date.

As with all medical consultations and procedures, you might like to prepare a list of questions to ask in advance as it is so easy to forget or not feel able to ask when you are there.

How is the examination done?

The nurse will help you onto a special couch with padded rests for your legs so that you are seated with your legs apart. You will be asked to remove your underwear, so you might like to wear a skirt. If your legs are uncovered, a towel or sheet is put across your knees so that as little as possible of your body is exposed. As when you have your cervical screening at your GP's surgery, it feels very undignified – but remember, the staff are well accustomed to the procedure and will help you feel comfortable.

The clinic environment is made as welcoming as possible and there may be posters and pictures on the walls and perhaps music to listen to. The nurse will be there all the time to talk to you if you wish and will make sure you are alright.

The doctor uses a speculum, the same instrument that was used during the screening, to enable them to see your cervix. They may apply a substance such as dilute acetic acid that causes any abnormal cells to change to a white appearance, making them more easy to see. If no abnormal area is detected on application of acetic acid, iodine may be applied to the cervix to highlight abnormalities which are invisible to normal light inspection.

If abnormal cells are seen, a small sample (a biopsy) may be taken. This is not normally painful but you may be offered a local anaesthetic if a larger sample is needed. If you are concerned, or if you feel pain afterwards, medical advice is that you can use paracetamol as a pain-killer but it is best not to take aspirin or ibuprofen as these substances may increase the risk of bleeding (your GP will be able to provide further advice).

You may experience a slight discharge after the procedure, especially if a biopsy is taken. If this does not stop after a few days or you have any bleeding, it is best to see your GP.

Treatment for pre-cancerous changes

Pre-cancerous changes are classified differently once they have been diagnosed using a biopsy. In chapter 3 we said that the results of your cervical screening may be described as showing mild, moderate or severe dyskaryosis. This term simply describes what the cells taken in your sample look like under the microscope, i.e. that they have abnormal nuclei.

When a sample of tissue is taken during a biopsy, it is possible to make a more accurate diagnosis of the degree of abnormality of the cells and whether they show any pre-cancerous changes, or whether cancer cells are actually developing.

'The cervix is covered by a layer of cells (similar to those of the skin) called squamous epithelium.'

The CIN classification of pre-cancerous changes

The term used in this classification is CIN, which is short for cervical intra-epithelial neoplasia. CIN is not cancer, but CIN cells can sometimes become cancerous. The websites and books listed at the back of this book can give you information to various degrees of detail depending on how much medical description you feel like reading, but here is a simple overview.

The cervix is covered by a layer of cells (similar to those of the skin) called squamous epithelium.

In basic terms, CIN classifications are:

- CIN 1 – the cells in the lower third of the epithelium are abnormal. You may be offered treatment or your consultant may advise that you wait and see if the cells return to normal.

- CIN 2 – the cells in the lower two thirds of the epithelium are abnormal. In this case, you will usually be offered treatment as described below.

- CIN 3 – here the cells in the full thickness of the epithelium are abnormal and you will usually require treatment to help the cells return to normal.

In summary, CIN responds to treatment and any level of CIN may, and often does, go away spontaneously.

Treatment at the colposcopy clinic

Some treatments of abnormal cells can be done at the clinic. In some cases, you may have the treatment and the biopsy at the same time.

For example, my cervical smear showed severe dyskaryosis and therefore instead of simply an examination, I was treated by a loop diathermy (also known as large loop excision of the transformation zone or LLETZ) which removed some tissue that could be analysed. This procedure often removes all the abnormal cells so that sometimes no further treatment is required. In my case, the tissue removed showed not only CIN 3 but invasive cancer cells, which is why I was given further treatment as will be explained in later chapters.

Types of treatment

There are various types of treatment that you may have at the colposcopy clinic.

Large loop excision of the transformation zone (LLETZ)
This is the most common form of treatment in the UK. The area of the cervix containing the abnormal cells is cut out using a loop of wire heated by an electric current. The heat also seals the area and reduces bleeding.

The procedure is carried out under local anaesthetic – in other words, the anaesthetic which numbs the area is applied directly in a similar way to when you have a filling at the dentist.

You should not feel pain at the time, but it may feel uncomfortable. You might feel a little strange afterwards, a bit like having a tooth out when you may feel a bit wobbly. It is, after all, a type of surgery even though it's a minor procedure. The letter you receive may advise you to bring someone with you who can drive you home, which is well worth considering.

For a few days afterwards, you may feel pain similar to period pain and possibly light bleeding or a discharge. You will be advised not to use tampons or to have sex for three weeks. A phone number will be given to you in case you have any worries or questions.

Laser treatments

This is different technology but is used in a similar way to the LLETZ procedure to remove abnormal cells and take a sample for analysis.

Less common methods

These include cryotherapy which freezes the abnormal cells to destroy them and cold coagulation which still uses heat but at a lower temperature (lower than used in the LLETZ procedure) to destroy the cells. These methods do not allow a sample of tissue to be analysed.

You may have heard of a method called cone biopsy. It is not usually performed nowadays. Instead, if a more extensive excision is required, the colposcopist performs an LLETZ followed by a 'top hat'. This is another deeper loop excision.

Talking to your GP or consultant

As soon as you are called for a cervical screening (smear) test, you may have questions and concerns. However, it can be difficult to pluck up courage to ask questions; you may feel that the GP, nurse or consultant is busy, or you may be embarrassed (especially with a delicate subject such as difficulties to do with sex and your 'private parts').

However, the medical professionals you encounter are just that – professionals – and they are all trained to talk to you and to answer your questions. Remember though, they cannot read your mind so cannot guess at every possible question you may have, so please ask – there is no such thing as a stupid question, nothing is too trivial if it is a concern for you!

Tactics to help

There are various things you can do to make sure you get all the information you need when you see your GP or consultant:

- Take a list of questions with you in a notebook and write down the answers as you go along.

- If you think of something else at any time, jot it down quickly so you don't forget.

- Ask the person you are seeing to repeat anything you don't understand or explain in different words. Medical terms are second nature to doctors and it is important that they are used as they have very precise meanings – but it is not always obvious to people not medically trained what they mean.

- Take someone with you if you can, and ask them to take notes and listen carefully for you.

'Ask the person you are seeing to repeat anything you don't understand or explain in different words.'

Information

You should be offered information in writing, leaflets etc., and if English is not your first language these will be available in a format that is best for you. Information should be available in large print, audio format or Braille. You should also be given a phone number in case you think of any questions after you have left the consultation.

Remember too that your GP can help and there is also the help list in the back of this book.

It is important to emphasise that the very best source of information is your own consultant or specialist nurse. Your particular case, treatment and reasons for being offered that particular treatment will be unique to you. General information – such as that offered here, in other books and on websites, or through talking to other patients – is just that; it's general, not specific to you, so please talk to your GP, nurse or consultant.

Pregnancy and an abnormal cervical screening test result

If you have treatment for abnormal cells, there can be a small risk of a premature birth. Research also shows that this appears to increase with the amount of tissue that is removed. Your GP will know about this from your medical records and, as always, you should discuss any concerns that you have with them.

If you receive an abnormal cervical screening result while you are pregnant, you will not normally be offered any treatment until after your baby is born. In *Preventing Cervical Cancer*, Dr Anne Szarewski says:

'Fortunately, the vast majority of abnormalities can safely be left for nine months until the baby has been safely delivered. Remember that the cells take a long time to develop through all the stages of abnormality to actual cancer.' (p. 69)

If you are told that you have CIN 1, 2 or 3, it is also unlikely that treatment will be suggested until after the birth. These changes are pre-cancerous and do not mean that you have cervical cancer. You may be asked to attend a colposcopy treatment so the consultant can keep an eye on what is happening.

If you are told that you have cervical cancer during pregnancy, there will be some difficult decisions to make. You will need to discuss all the options with your doctor. As Dr Szarewski says: 'ultimately, it is you and your partner who have to live with the consequences of any decision you reach, so you need to have thought about it very carefully' (*Preventing Cervical Cancer*, p. 69).

Summing Up

This chapter has described the follow-up you may be offered if you receive an abnormal result from a cervical screening test. It cannot be emphasised too often that this result does not mean that you have cancer; it simply means abnormal changes have occurred. Even if further investigations at a colposcopy clinic discover you have cells with CIN 1, 2 or 3 changes, these are still pre-cancerous and will most probably respond to treatment.

You have also been given some information about the terms you may hear used if you are given a diagnosis of cervical cancer. Don't worry if, like me, you find this all too much to take in – you can ask your consultant, GP or nurse to repeat and explain any parts of your specific diagnosis that you wish to understand better. There is also a glossary at the back of this book listing some of the medical terms you may come across.

5

Treatment for Cervical Cancer

This chapter will cover all the different treatments that you may be offered if you are diagnosed with cervical cancer. As always, everyone's situation is unique to them, and your particular treatment may be different to the experiences of others.

The type of treatment that you will be offered will be discussed with you. You may be given a choice, and it is likely that your consultant will recommend which course of action they think is best. It is a choice, and you do not have to take their advice. If you wish, you can ask for time to consider the options and you are entitled to ask for a second opinion.

Your consultant will talk to colleagues and they will either meet you or be available for questions. For example, in my case, I was informed that the best option was surgery. The consultant I saw was a gynaecological surgery specialist, and she outlined the reasons for the recommendation and stated that she had already discussed my case with her colleagues in the oncology department (responsible for chemotherapy and radiotherapy treatments).

Stages and grades of cancer

You may hear these two terms used, and I found it quite confusing, especially when I had just got to grips with the types of dyskaryosis for abnormal cells and the CIN terms for pre-cancerous cells.

They all describe different things though, so it will be useful to explain these distinctions very briefly.

This information is also available on a number of the health information websites mentioned in the help list. These are also excellent places to find the most up-to-date information written in clear and easily understandable language.

'The stage of a cancer describes its size and whether it has moved. The grade explains how quickly it may develop.'

Stages

This term refers to the size of the cancer and whether it has moved.

- Stage 1 – cancer cells are only found within the cervix.
- Stage 2 – cancer cells are found in the upper part of the vagina or surrounding tissues.
- Stage 3 – cancer cells have spread further into the pelvis, the lymph nodes or the lower part of the vagina.
- Stage 4 – when cancer cells have spread to the bladder, bowel or beyond the pelvis.

Grades

This term explains how quickly the cancer can develop. A biopsy will determine the grade of cancer.

- Grade 1 – low grade, slow growing and less likely to spread.
- Grade 2 – moderate grade, the cells are slightly faster growing and look more abnormal.

- Grade 3 – high grade, likely to be faster spreading, cells grow more quickly and look very abnormal under the microscope.

Once doctors know the stage and grade of your cancer, the best treatment can be decided. For more information on this, please visit www.macmillan.org.uk. If you follow the links to 'cancer type', 'cervical cancer' and then to 'staging and grading', you will find more details and advice to help you.

Please do not feel you have to remember all these distinctions – your consultant will explain to you anything that refers to your own diagnosis and should give you information to take away with you if appropriate. Do ask as many questions as you wish so you are sure that you are clear about what you are being told and what it means for your decisions on treatment.

Surgery

Depending on the location and spread of your cancer, surgery may be the first option. Fortunately, cervical cancer is one type of cancer that can be totally removed if treated early enough. For this reason, it is vital that women attend cervical screening appointments when invited by their GP.

As discussed earlier in the section on treatment for an abnormal result (chapter 4), some treatments can be carried out in the colposcopy clinic as an outpatient. However, if the cancer cells have begun to spread, or there is any suspicion of this, you may be advised to have a hysterectomy.

Hysterectomy

This is removal of the womb in most cases, but sometimes part of the vagina, nearby lymph nodes and the ovaries can be removed as well.

If possible, the surgeon will avoid removing the ovaries, particularly in younger women as removal will result in an early menopause. However, if this is necessary, you may be able to receive hormone replacement therapy (HRT) to avoid the onset of menopause until you are the age when this would happen naturally.

The type of hysterectomy where lymph nodes are removed is known as a Wertheim's hysterectomy. It is a much bigger operation than a simple hysterectomy and this affects the time it may take you to recover. The reason for removing lymph nodes is that the spread of cancer cells can take place through the lymph system. Checking the lymph nodes can help determine how far the cancer has spread (the stage), and aid a decision on whether you will need radiotherapy.

Trachelectomy

This is a special type of surgery that means that the ovaries and womb are not removed, so it may still be possible for a woman to have a baby.

However, this surgery is only suitable for women with very early stage cervical cancer. If you were to fall pregnant following a trachelectomy, there would be risks of miscarriage and the baby would have to be delivered by Caesarean section. You would also have to be referred to a specialist hospital – therefore, it would be important to discuss the benefits and risks with your doctor before considering this operation.

Preparing for surgery

When you receive a diagnosis of cancer and are told you need to have a major operation, it is a big shock to come to terms with. Everyone will react differently and sometimes treating yourself to some favourite things before you go into hospital can help you deal with the shock.

My list of treats included:

- Special outings, walks and spending time with friends.
- Time by myself when I didn't have to think about anyone else's feelings.
- Choosing favourite books to take into hospital (my choices included childhood favourites such as The Secret Garden and The Hobbit – comforting and easy to read).

Of course, your list will be different to my examples, and after surgery you will be advised to take things easy for a while so if you are a very active person, you may want to do some of those favourite things before surgery – whether it is running, cycling, mountain climbing or sky diving!

Being as fit as possible before surgery is a good thing of course; if a person is very overweight, it is common for doctors to advise weight loss before surgery. However, you will have a chance to discuss your particular circumstances with your consultant if necessary.

Recovering from surgery

When you leave hospital after your surgery, you will be given information leaflets and advice on what you can do and how soon. For example, it is usually recommended that you don't try to drive until at least six weeks after abdominal surgery such as a hysterectomy.

You will also be advised to be careful when lifting and pushing things – even examples such as not lifting a full kettle or doing the ironing to start with. If you were the person who always did everything at home, it can be difficult for you not to go straight back to doing this. It may also be hard for other people to realise that you will need help.

It might be helpful to discuss with your family the expected recovery time and what your GP recommends you should and shouldn't do during this period. Perhaps give them some leaflets to read or point them to websites, such as Macmillan Cancer Support, so they can see for themselves what the specialists recommend. There is a balance between gradually becoming more active and regaining your fitness and doing too much which could delay your recovery.

Side effects

How individuals are affected by the surgery varies. Not only will the actual process of the operation be different – for example, you may have more or fewer lymph nodes removed than someone else – but we all vary in how our bodies recover.

You may find it takes longer than you expect and you may experience post-operative pain. This, for me, was the main side effect and was a result of the surgery rather than the cancer itself. But the surgery saved my life, so that is always in the back of my mind. You will be given pain-killing medication if required and this is something to keep talking to your GP about if necessary.

Other side effects may include constipation, particularly early after the operation, but you will probably be given medication to help with this. You may also feel some changes in the way your bladder works; it may be hard to empty when you go to the bathroom and you may find you have stress incontinence – slight leaks when you cough, sneeze or laugh. You can ask your GP for advice on this and there are exercises you can learn to strengthen the muscles in this area.

Your sex life will be another area of life that's affected. Your partner may be very concerned about hurting you and after surgery you will be advised not to have sex for at least six weeks. However, it will be important for both of you to talk about this and

'It might be helpful to discuss with your family the expected recovery time and what your GP recommends you should and shouldn't do during this period.'

to continue to feel connected intimately with each other. Lots of cuddles can help in reassuring you that you are still loved and cared for, and there are also ways of touching and loving each other that can be satisfying while you are still recovering from the surgery. It is important that you both feel comfortable with the decision to begin a sexual relationship after surgery, so communication is vital between you and your partner.

There is good advice and information available online, for example the Macmillan Cancer Support website has a section on sexuality. Chapter 6 of this book has more on emotions and feelings.

Radiotherapy

Radiotherapy is used to treat cancer by bombarding the cancer cells with high-energy rays that destroy them. Over the years, better and better treatments have been developed that are able to target the cancer cells more precisely and affect the healthy cells less.

You will be offered radiotherapy if the cancer has spread beyond the area where it can be removed by surgery, or the treatment could be given after surgery if there is a risk that the cancer may have spread. Radiotherapy may also be given in combination with chemotherapy (see later in this chapter).

Types of radiotherapy

Two types of radiotherapy can be used: external and internal, and you may be offered both. You will be asked to one or more appointments with your cancer specialist (known as a clinical oncologist) which will be to plan your treatment. You will have marks put on your skin so that the radiotherapist can line up the beam to the precise place to repeat the treatment every time.

Unfortunately, radiotherapy will stop the ovaries working and will produce an early menopause in young women.

External radiotherapy

This is given as a short daily treatment over a period of weeks, which will vary according to your individual treatment plan. Before each treatment, the radiotherapist will position you on the couch and leave the room but you will be able to talk to them if you wish. You have to lie very still for a few minutes.

Most people find it is the daily journey to the hospital that is most wearing. After a while you may experience some side effects such as nausea and you may be given medication to help reduce this. You may find it hard to eat properly but it's important to maintain a healthy diet and drink plenty of fluids. You might find it easier to eat little and often.

Delia, who I interviewed for *Flying in the Face of Fear*, said:

'The first few sessions of radiotherapy went well and I felt no side effects. As days went on, the treatment took its toll. By the end of the three weeks I couldn't make the 20 minute journey without a sick bag.'

The support of friends made a great difference to Delia and she describes how every day a different person would arrive on the doorstep to drive her to hospital. Her friends had worked out a rota to take the pressure off Delia's husband.

Internal radiotherapy (brachytherapy)

Due to the position of the cervix, it is possible to give very targeted radiotherapy by placing the sources of the radiation actually inside the body.

This means a stronger dose can be given (with less damage to other tissues of the body) which may be more effective in destroying the cancer cells. To do this, tubes containing radioactive material are placed inside your body while you are under a general anaesthetic. You have to stay isolated from other people for several days as the radioactivity could be harmful to them and you also have to lie very still.

It can be a very lonely and sad time but it is only for a short while. The removal of the tubes can be a painful process but you will be given pain-killers to help with this.

Side effects

After radiotherapy you will need to rest and build up your strength again. You will probably feel very tired and sometimes nauseous, but you can ask your GP for medicines to help control sickness or diarrhoea.

As well as the effects mentioned during treatment, you may have soreness or redness of the skin in the area that has been given external radiotherapy. It is advisable to avoid scented soaps and creams for a while as they may irritate the skin further.

'The first few sessions of radiotherapy went well and I felt no side effects. As days went on, the treatment took its toll. By the end of the three weeks I couldn't make the 20 minute journey without a sick bag.'

Radiotherapy may cause narrowing of the vagina that can make sexual intercourse painful. As discussed in the section on surgery, your partner can help by being aware and sympathetic, so communication between you both is essential. You may also be given dilators to be used regularly to help widen the vagina gradually over time. There is more information on this in chapter 7.

Some women may experience longer term effects such as damage to the bowel, bladder or lymphoedema. Lymphoedema is swelling in the legs when the lymph glands in the pelvis have been affected by radiotherapy (or sometimes by surgery) which is caused by the lymph fluid collecting.

Everyone is affected differently by their treatment. If you become worried about side effects, there is specialist advice available to help you avoid and deal with them; in the first instance contact your GP for advice.

Late effects of radiotherapy

Very few people suffer from what is called 'the late effects' of treatment. This means a side effect that does not happen until some time after you have finished radiotherapy. See also chapter 7 for more information.

Chemotherapy

This is the use of drugs to destroy the cancer cells in the body. They are sometimes given intravenously (injected by a drip into a vein) or by taking tablets.

Chemotherapy may be used before surgery or radiotherapy to shrink the cancer before these types of treatments are undertaken. It may also be used at the same time as radiotherapy as it is thought to make the radiotherapy treatment more effective.

In cases where the cancer is more advanced, or has returned after other treatments, chemotherapy may be given to try to control the spread of the cancer, shrink the tumour and give a better quality of life.

Side effects

Hair loss

The side effect of chemotherapy that everyone has heard of, and probably fears most, is losing your hair. Particularly for women, hair is such an important part of who you are and how you see yourself that it can be devastating to even contemplate losing it.

Please remember though – there are ways of dealing with it and you will choose the best option for you. Some people cut their hair very short before they start losing it so it is less of a shock then; some people are happy to show their head with no hair; others choose to use scarves or wigs. Once again, there are organisations and places to help you with this issue. For example, Macmillan Cancer Support has a page devoted to this with all sorts of information, including financial help and how to have fun with different styles.

Lack of appetite

As with radiotherapy, you may experience nausea, vomiting and lack of appetite. These can lead to anaemia and weight loss. You may also experience a sore mouth that adds to these problems. There are liquid meals that you can buy or prepare for yourself and you will be given advice on this.

Summing Up

The descriptions above sound formidable, and the treatments are designed to fight a life-threatening disease. However, they only go on for a certain length of time and the side effects will wear off once treatment is complete.

Sometimes the emotional effects are the hardest to deal with, so the next chapter will look at these, offering advice and suggestions to help you cope.

During these times, you may well discover just how mentally strong you are and, in developing your own coping techniques that work for you and with the support you receive from family, friends and professionals, you will emerge a changed person.

Many people I have spoken to have said that although they wouldn't say they are glad they had cancer, they can declare that some of the changes to come out of it have been extremely positive.

Emotions and Feelings

The subject of abnormal smears and possible cancer is bound to bring up strong feelings and powerful emotions. Sometimes these can be overwhelming and in this chapter you will find some ideas for help and support if you are diagnosed with cancer. If it is a member of your family or a friend who is affected, you will have your own feelings to deal with as well as helping them.

There is a lot of support out there, whether you want to talk to someone on the phone, join an online group or go along to a meeting (or all of those things at different times). Even if none of these appeal to you, just knowing they are available can be a comfort in itself. One of the best places to start is Macmillan Cancer Support, either their website or the helpline. The help list in this book gives contact details for sources of information and support that you may find useful.

Dealing with my feelings

Everyone will have different reactions to bad news about their health. The first reaction might be shock, followed by denial ('this can't be happening to me!'), anger, sadness, anxiety and even depression for some people.

You may also feel relief at being given a diagnosis. If you have been worried about something being wrong, it may feel better to know exactly what that is, and to feel that you can now get on and do something about it.

There are many excellent sources of advice and help online. One that I used is Cancerbackup, which is now part of Macmillan Cancer Support. Follow the links to 'cancer information', then 'emotional effects', and you will find a variety of information.

When I was told I had an abnormal cervical screening test result in March 1994, I was not overly worried. But later in May I received the diagnosis of cancer from my GP. My first question was 'can I talk to someone else who has been through this?' My GP's reply was that she could not give me any names due to confidentiality. I am pleased to say that things have moved on a lot since then and it is easier to find local and national support groups and online groups where you can talk to other patients.

There are lots of suggestions in the help list at the back of this book. For example, Jo's Trust is a charity dedicated to helping people with cervical cancer. They have an online forum, a facility where you can ask questions of medical experts and receive a confidential reply, and they also hold regular 'Let's Meet' days. Another organisation, Health Talk Online (previously called DIPEx), has interviews with patients about all aspects of their experience.

The next thing I did was contact Cancerbackup (now part of Macmillan Cancer Support) and talk to the nurses on their helpline, who were enormously supportive. No question was too silly for them; they were calm and caring and were not upset by anything I might have said. You don't need to have a cancer diagnosis to call them, even if you have worries or concerns they will be able to help.

Your feelings if you are supporting someone else

If you are the family or a friend of someone who has received a cancer diagnosis, your feelings are equally important. Be aware that you will also feel shock, denial, anger, anxiety and all of those feelings usually associated with traumatic circumstances. It's a difficult time for everyone involved but try to remain positive; if you feel you're not coping please see your GP in the first instance and bear in mind that the Macmillan Cancer Support helpline caters for anyone affected by cancer.

Telling family and friends

The first thing you may have to do is to tell your close family about your diagnosis. My experience was that this was one of the hardest things of all. My closest family were of course most affected, but at least they knew that I had been for the colposcopy and biopsy.

You may find, like me, that after a while you just can't face making another phone call to break bad news to a friend. This is one example of where the friends who may say 'just let me know if there is anything I can do to help' really can help. You could ask each of them to ring specific people on your behalf to break the news.

One thing that surprised me was how I immediately felt as if I was no longer 'Mary' but 'a person with cancer' and everyone started to treat me differently. I also felt very responsible for other people's feelings and found myself trying to protect them.

You will probably find that you need someone who you can talk to openly about how you are feeling. However much you try, you won't be able to 'be positive' all the time as people may tell you (with the best of intentions). This is when it can be invaluable to talk to a counsellor, one of the helplines or to a really trusted friend who will simply allow you to feel and say exactly what you want and not try to 'fix' things.

A friend of mine recently said that she needed to think and express her negative thoughts to someone who wouldn't get upset to enable her to deal with them. She found that facing up to the worst that could happen, expressing any negative thoughts without well-meaning people saying 'you must be positive', helped her cope with other people's feelings about her illness.

Children

Telling children is one of the hardest parts of all when you have a diagnosis of any serious illness. Not only what to tell them but when and how much information to give them needs to be decided, perhaps in discussion with your partner and other close family.

Professional advice is that it is best to be as open as you can with children as appropriate for their age – or rather, as appropriate for their understanding, as this can vary. Children are perceptive and may know something is wrong even if you tell them nothing. If they feel they are being kept in the dark, they may worry and imagine the worst – which we all do at times.

Explain words simply, and use words that they will hear anyway like cancer. NHS Choices say:

'Explain it in language your children will understand. The word cancer becomes less frightening for everyone if it's described as cells that have grown faster than other cells in the body.'
(© NHS Choices: www.nhs.uk, accessed 19 August 2009.)

'The word cancer becomes less frightening for everyone if it's described as cells that have grown faster than other cells in the body.'
NHS Choices.

Not their fault

Children can often think that a parent being ill is their fault or a punishment for something they have done wrong. Make it clear for them that this is not true – explain that sometimes people get ill; it is not their fault, it is just bad luck, and all the doctors and nurses are doing their best to help Mummy get better.

Teenagers

Older children and teenagers may like to read information online when they feel like it. The US National Cancer Institute has a big range of booklets that you can view online or print if you wish – see the help list for details. Young people may also benefit from talking to someone outside the family, like a health professional, teacher or youth worker.

Employers and colleagues

A practical issue is telling people at work. Depending on your situation, you may or may not need time away from work. If you do, you will of course have to inform your employer through the usual procedures.

It is up to you to decide who you wish to tell outside the immediate requirements of your job role. People you work with should respect your wishes on this. My personal way of dealing with it was to tell my manager and ask her to inform the rest of my colleagues. I worked in a small company at the time and this was the best course of action for me.

If you work in a big organisation, this might not work for you, or in any case you may want to let as few people as possible know. It is entirely up to you.

Counselling and complementary therapies

As well as the help of your medical team, there are a lot of other things you can do to support yourself.

Counselling

You may find it useful to talk to someone outside the family who is not emotionally involved with your situation. Your GP, consultant and nurses can help, and it may also be useful to talk to a counsellor. This service should be available through your GP, and if you are close to a cancer information centre they may have counsellors who specialise in working with cancer patients.

My experience was that I didn't need to speak to someone straightaway but I found counselling useful after I had been discharged from hospital. As always, everyone's situation is different, so it is important to access whatever support is useful for you.

Complementary therapies

Many people find that using complementary therapies of various kinds can help them deal with the symptoms of their illness, the side effects of the treatment and the emotional issues. A very important benefit is that these therapies tend to encourage you to relax deeply in a peaceful and safe environment, and that in itself can be very beneficial.

Many cancer support centres and groups provide free sessions to their members. Therapies such as massage, reflexology, meditation, reiki, acupuncture and aromatherapy might be available in your area. Or you may prefer to find your own practitioner by recommendation from friends and pay privately.

'If you are supporting a family member with cancer, you have your own emotions and feelings to deal with.'

How to help someone in my family

As mentioned earlier, if you are supporting a family member with cancer, you will have your own emotions and feelings to deal with, plus the added worry of the unknown future and day-to-day issues.

Practical matters

Anne Orchard, who wrote a book and started the web community Families Facing Cancer (see help list), suggests various actions that the patient and their close family can take.

For example, she suggests sitting down together and writing a list of all the practical things that friends could help with:

'This helps you to be ready when someone asks to help, and it also helps you to determine any items that the person with cancer deems too private – so you can designate those items only to the closest family members. For example, your cancer patient may be quite happy to have others sit with them so that family members can get a break – but they may not be comfortable accepting assistance from others at meal times if they require help with the basics of eating. Some tasks that others can easily help with include:

- Laundry.
- Meal preparation.
- Trips to the pharmacy.
- Dog walking.
- Running other errands.
- Garden maintenance.
- House cleaning.

'If you're a primary caregiver for someone with cancer, be ready to say "yes" when others offer to help. If their offers are not specific, you can keep in mind their talents and time availability when making requests. Is a church member a seamstress? Have her mend clothes and take in those that have become too big.'
(© Families Facing Cancer, www.familiesfacingcancer.org/lessons, accessed 5 December 2009).

There is plenty more practical advice on the website, plus a forum where you can contact people in a similar situation to yourself. Well worth a visit!

Look after yourself too

You will need to be aware of your own health and wellbeing. It may feel selfish, but how can you do your best for them if you are stressed and become unwell yourself?

The things we discussed in chapter 2 about life balance are relevant here. You will need your own support away from the person who has cancer, time to enjoy at least some of your usual activities – whether it's getting some exercise and fresh air, or talking to your friends.

Summing Up

The word cancer is guaranteed to provoke fear and negative feelings. Thinking of it very simply, as advised when talking to children, will help adults too – for example, cancer cells have simply grown faster than other cells in the body.

Acknowledging your feelings, whether negative or positive, and getting as much support as possible will help you cope, whether you are the person with the cancer diagnosis or someone whose family or friend is experiencing this.

The help list will give you details of some of the many sources of help and support available.

7

After Treatment

This chapter will talk about the time immediately after your treatment finishes, and chapter 8 about life after cancer. For some people, this is life with cancer, as modern treatments enable many people to live for many years with cancer as a chronic disease.

Medical follow up

As discussed in chapter 5, when you first leave hospital after surgery or complete your radiotherapy or chemotherapy treatment, there will be a period of time when you are recovering from the immediate effects of the treatment.

After this you will be asked to return to hospital or a local clinic regularly for follow-up appointments. If you have surgery, you will probably be given an appointment six weeks after your operation.

The frequency of check-ups will depend on your individual treatment, speed of recovery and the policy in the area where you live. Usually appointments are at three months, then every six months and then annual. After five years you will probably be officially discharged from the care of the consultant.

Support and someone to talk to

Professional support

'I found the best thing was talking to friends, and being a "buddy" visiting other women to support them after their treatment.'

Shani, cervical cancer patient.

While you are having regular follow-up appointments, it is a good time to take the opportunity to continue making lists of any questions you have so you can ask the doctor while you are there.

You will be given a contact number for your gynaecological support nurse, and they will be available to talk about any worries or concerns that you have. Do not feel that you are being a nuisance if you call them; it is recognised that this type of support makes a big difference to people's recovery.

Helplines such as Macmillan Cancer Support are also available. Once you start feeling better physically, you may also feel you would like to join a local support group. The Macmillan Cancer Support website has a search facility for groups in your area, and there is also an online forum (see help list).

Jo's Trust, also mentioned previously, is an excellent resource for women who have had cervical cancer. As well as events and an online forum, the website has a feature where you can ask a question that is sent to medical specialists who provide private, confidential advice for you. As mentioned above, the first place to ask about your treatment is your own GP, nurse or consultant as they will know all the details of your particular case. However, having access to a second source of expert information is very useful and reassuring.

Friends and family

During your treatment, you might not feel like seeing friends as much as you used to, so after treatment is a time when you can pick up these contacts again and arrange some treats together. Meeting up for coffee or lunch, a walk in a park or the countryside – these will be milestones in your path back to fitness and a normal life. Chatting to friends or family who know what you have been through will be a support and also a distraction for you from any lingering worries that may be in the back of your mind.

Accepting changes

Most, if not all, people who have had cancer find that this is always with them and something that becomes part of their life (see chapter 8 for more information).

Change always happens in life anyway, whether we like it or not. Sometimes this is hard to accept, especially when there is loss involved. If you are treated for cervical cancer, you may lose your fertility and the chance of having children in the future. Even if this is not an issue for you, many women feel they need time to grieve for the loss of a part of them that makes them a woman.

Chapter 6 dealt in detail with emotions and feelings and of course these will continue to be affected after your treatment ends.

You may find that some of these activities can help:

- Listing things that have changed, without judging them 'good' or 'bad'.
- Writing a gratitude list of people and things you are thankful for.
- Writing, painting, drawing, making models, or doing any other creative activity.
- Spending time outside in nature, noticing all the little things usually taken for granted.

Getting back to normal

You may feel at some stages that life will never be the same again and, of course, in some ways it will not. Some of this is in a positive way; you may find that the experience of having cancer renews and increases your appreciation of all the good things in your life.

Physical recovery takes time and your doctors will recommend what physical activities you undertake at certain stages. There is a balance between not over-doing things and making sure you continue to progress and feel able to increase what you can do.

You may find that you feel very tired and need more rest even after your treatment has finished. It will be useful to keep a diary or journal so you can note the times of day when you feel best and most able to do things, and the times when you need to rest.

When it comes to recovering from a serious illness with the treatment of surgery and/ or radiotherapy and/or chemotherapy, there is much to be gained from the expression 'pacing yourself.'

Macmillan Cancer Support run courses that will help you with this. There is one called 'New Perspectives' where you can learn ways of managing your recovery. Macmillan are also developing a 'self-management toolkit' which will include mini-workshops covering areas such as relaxation, exercise, healthy eating, communication, sex and body image. These sessions are intended to develop personal confidence and the skills to address the day-to-day issues of living with and beyond cancer.

The details of the latest workshops and programmes run by Macmillan can be found in the Learn Zone area of their website (see help list).

Other ideas and information can be found through local support groups and in some of the books mentioned in the book list on page 91.

Sex and relationships

One of the difficult aspects of cervical cancer is that it affects such a personal area of your body.

Earlier chapters have mentioned some of the side effects of treatments. Both surgery and radiotherapy can alter how your vagina feels to you and to your partner during intercourse.

If you have radiotherapy, it will be suggested that you use a set of dilators. These are plastic cones that you put inside your vagina to stretch it.

Shani says very frankly: 'I would like to stress that after the treatment do use the dilators, in spite of any pain and discomfort. And take the advice given; start to attempt a physical relationship with your partner as soon as possible – within 18 months I was OK.'

There will be advice and support available from your gynaecological specialist nurse, so although you may be embarrassed at first, do ask for any help you need. You will also be able to access support for your partner, either together or individually – whichever is right for the two of you and your circumstances.

Living with cancer

Late effects of radiotherapy

Very few people suffer from what is called 'the late effects' of treatment. This means a side effect that may not happen until some time after radiotherapy is finished.

The Cancer Help UK website has a very helpful and clear section on this, where it is explained:

'Generally, radiotherapy can cause body tissues to become tighter and less elastic. Doctors call this fibrosis. This can have some lasting effects, depending on the part of the body being treated. It can cause thickening of the skin in the treatment area, for example. Everyone treated will have changes to the ovaries, womb and vagina. But you may not have other lasting effects from radiotherapy. If you do get any, they can come on months or even years after your treatment finishes. Some people may have swelling in their legs (lymphoedema) or bladder and bowel side effects.'
(Taken from CancerHelp UK, the patient information website of Cancer Research UK: www.cancerhelp.org.uk, accessed 5 December 2009.)

It is important to remember that these side effects are rare and currently it is not possible to say why some women experience them and others do not. Cancer Research UK continually conducts research in all areas of cancer and its treatment to help discover more about these side effects and ways of avoiding them.

Advanced cancer

When you are first diagnosed with cancer, it will be natural to fear the worst and worry about it spreading to other parts of your body. As has been emphasised throughout this book, ways of preventing cervical cancer are being developed all the time, and if you do develop it, the ways of treating it are becoming more and more successful.

However, it is possible that you may be told you have advanced cancer. This does not necessarily mean that it has spread widely; it can be from stage 2 onwards where the cancer has spread outside the cervix (see chapter 5 for information on staging and grading cancer).

Whether the cancer can be treated will depend on how far it has spread, how much cancer there is and exactly where it has spread to.

Even if your cervical cancer comes back after your first treatment, it may still be possible to cure it using radiotherapy, chemotherapy, surgery or a combination of these treatments. Everyone's treatment is different as your particular condition will be different. Exactly what treatment you are offered will depend on the treatment you have already had as well as the spread and location of the cancer cells.

More advanced or terminal cancer

If your cancer spreads to other parts of your body (known as secondary cancer or metastasis), a cure will not be possible. However, you will be offered treatment to control the symptoms of your cancer. The treatment may slow down the spread of the cancer or control pain by shrinking tumours that are pressing on nerves.

Cancer Help UK has an excellent section on the treatments available for advanced and terminal cancer, as does Macmillan Cancer Support. You will want to look at all the options and discuss with your doctor and your family before you make a decision on whether to go for further treatment.

Some people live with cancer for many years with a good quality of life and, depending on their age and other factors, they may in fact die of something unrelated rather than their cancer.

However, for some people the prospect of the end of life has to be faced. Of course, none of us actually know when this will be, but realising that it probably will be within a certain period of time can be difficult.

If you, or someone you love, is in this situation, there are a number of ways to help you feel in control. As well as the treatment to deal with the effects of the cancer, you might wish to do some of these things:

'Some people live with cancer for many years with a good quality of life.'

- Write letters for loved ones to read after your death.

- Make 'memory boxes' with special things for people you love.

- Write letters for your children to read at special stages in their lives (e.g birthdays and Christmas, leaving school). You will think of lots of occasions when you would like them to feel that you are with them even if you cannot be in reality.

- Visit the local hospice in case you want to spend some time there. The staff are specially trained and hospices can often be a happy and uplifting place for someone dealing with advanced or terminal cancer.

- Put all your affairs in order so that you are not leaving extra things for your family to deal with.

- Plan your funeral – this may sound gloomy, but many people actually find this enjoyable in a way. You can choose the music you want, leave instructions for the type of service, say whether you would like people to wear traditional black or more brightly coloured clothes, etc.

While you are doing these things, you may find that it is sad and painful but also that it helps you think more clearly. Many people find that telling the people around them that you love them and giving them the chance to tell you back helps everyone feel less regretful about things they wished they had said before a person passes away.

There are a number of books and websites to help you with this process – you will find some of these in the help list. You may find that this is a time when you take up some professional help from a counsellor or bereavement specialist.

Summing Up

This chapter has ended on a rather serious note: it is necessary to face up to what could happen. You may find, as people have said to me, that once you face up to the worst then you can plan and live day-to-day enjoying your life.

The worst may not happen, or not for some time, and every day is precious. This is true for all of us and people often say that a diagnosis of cancer is a 'wake-up call' and empowers them to do what they really want in life.

It cannot be emphasised too often that you are not alone – there is a huge range of help and support out there. You can choose to take advantage of this, or choose not to – it is entirely up to you.

Many people do make a full recovery and find life returning to normal. Chapter 8 will look at life after cancer.

8

Life After Cancer

The many advances in treatments for cancer over recent years means that more and more people are coming out the other side and are living 'life after cancer'.

This chapter looks at some of the challenges and celebrations that this might bring for you. You may hear the term 'survivorship' used, which is about this experience of life after cancer or living with cancer as a chronic illness.

Chronic illness means a disease that does not kill you, so rather than a diagnosis of cancer meaning that you are almost certain to die, these days you are more likely to survive and have a good quality of life for many years afterwards.

Coping with physical changes

As mentioned in chapter 7, you may experience physical changes as a result of the treatment you receive for cervical cancer. Whether you have surgery or radiotherapy, it will almost certainly mean that you will no longer be able to have children.

If your ovaries are affected, it will also mean that you will experience a premature, and sudden, menopause. Normally women would go through this gradually as their ovaries produce less oestrogen and they may have the various side effects of this such as hot flushes and night sweats. You may be offered HRT to counteract this, if it is suitable for you.

Other physical effects such as pain from the operation or bladder or bowel problems may lessen with time. You may not believe it at first and it may take much longer than you hope or expect, but over time it is remarkable how our bodies can heal and adjust to the physical changes.

Dealing with emotional effects

You may find that during the period when you are undergoing treatment, you can focus on fighting the cancer and battling to beat the disease. You may also find that once your treatment has ended and you are discharged by your consultant after five or more years of being followed up, you feel almost lost.

If you have been diagnosed, you will already have been through an emotional rollercoaster. What may have kept you going might have been always focusing on the next stage whatever that was. So, when there isn't really a 'next stage', what do you do?

It could be that you will want to talk to someone else who has been through the experience, or you may want to ask for some professional help such as counselling. Although you may already have done this, it could also be very helpful at this stage.

People sometimes say 'I know I should be grateful I have survived, but…'. During treatment, you may find yourself so busy dealing with all the practical things that you forget to give yourself time to cope with the emotional effects. It can be important to allow yourself to grieve for the things you have lost: the parts of your body if you have had surgery; the chance to have children or add to your family.

If you feel that you want to have children, you may wish to explore the possibility of fostering or adoption at some time in the future. This is a big commitment and one you will want to discuss in depth with your partner and family and obtain as much professional advice on as you can. See *Adoption and Fostering – A Parent's Guide* (Need2Know) for further information.

The charitable organisation Adoption UK has a website with full information on the differing rules in England, Scotland, Wales and Northern Ireland, plus support and services such as message boards to share experiences.

Even though you may not look any different, physically losing your womb or losing your fertility through radiotherapy can have a huge impact on how you feel as a woman.

Everyone is different and will choose to do different things to help themselves through this. Some things that have helped other women include:

- Writing about feelings in a journal or diary.

- Using drawing or painting as a means of expression: it doesn't matter if you feel you are not 'artistic', the therapeutic benefit can be very powerful.

- Taking this one step further, working with a professional art therapist, either by yourself or in a group.

- Treating yourself to new outfits, make-up, even a professional make-over by an image consultant or colour advisor.

Local cancer support groups are a wonderful source of companionship and facilities such as art and crafts groups. They also often provide access to complementary therapies such as reflexology and aromatherapy that can help with relaxation and stress relief.

Getting back to work

When you were first diagnosed with cervical cancer, you will have decided who to tell at your workplace, whether that was only those that needed to know by law or others as well. Having been through all that and perhaps been away from work for some time, starting work again can seem like a major hurdle – it's also a big achievement and a milestone on your road to recovery.

Of course, everyone's situation is different. Employees with cancer have various legal rights that are explained very clearly on the Macmillan Cancer Support website.

Some people who are able, and wish to, literally work through their treatment, but for most people a complete break from work is necessary.

When you and your doctors feel you are ready to go back to work, you will probably wish to start gradually with part-time working. Many people find that they feel fatigued very quickly, this is a normal effect of cancer treatment, whether it is surgery, radiotherapy or chemotherapy (or any combination). So it is important not to take on too much and to build up over time.

You may find that it is best not to drive too much, and if so, you may be able to arrange to work some or all of your hours at home. With modern technology this is becoming a more and more accepted as a way of working anyway.

'Many people find that they feel fatigued very quickly – this is a normal effect of cancer treatment.'

Some people are not able to return to the work they did before they were diagnosed and this can be a difficult thing to come to terms with. As someone with cancer you may not consider yourself 'disabled' but you are protected by the Disability Discrimination Act (DDA) and other legislation.

The section below is drawn from the advice offered on the Macmillan Cancer Support website:

Everyone with cancer is classed as disabled under the DDA and so is protected by this Act. The DDA covers workers who were disabled in the past, even if they are no longer disabled. So a person who had a cancer in the past that has been successfully treated and is now 'cured' will still be covered by the DDA. This means their employer must not discriminate against them for a reason relating to their past cancer.

The employer has a duty to make 'reasonable adjustments' to workplaces and working practices to ensure that people with a disability are not at a disadvantage compared to others.

What is considered a 'reasonable adjustment' depends on things such as:

- the cost of making the adjustment
- the amount the adjustment will benefit the employee
- the practicality of making the adjustment
- whether making the adjustment will affect the employer's business/service/financial situation.

(Source: 'Work and Cancer' online publication accessed via

http://www.macmillan.org.uk/GetInvolved/Campaigns/WorkingThroughCancer/ WorkingThroughCancer.aspx accessed 6 December 2009)

Your employer is not allowed to discriminate against you because of your illness.

They have a duty to make to help you cope. Examples of 'reasonable adjustments' include:

- Allowing you time off for treatment and medical appointments.
- Allowing flexibility with working hours, the tasks you have to perform or your working environment.

The definition of what is 'reasonable' depends on the situation, for example, how much it would affect your employer's business.

It will help if you give your employer as much information as possible about how much time you will need off and when. Talk to your human resources department if you have one. Your union or staff association representative should also be able to give you advice.

If you are having difficulties with your employer, your union or your local Citizens Advice Bureau may be able to help. The Macmillan publication quoted above is also available as a booklet, full details are in the book list..

What if I am not able to go back to work?

Some people are not able to go back to work for a considerable time, if at all.

You may not be aware that there is financial support available while you are being treated for cancer and after your treatment has ended if you still require it. You will also be entitled to free subscriptions.

When you first start treatment, this may be the last thing on your mind, but as time goes on it can be a big source of worry and stress. There will be a social worker at the hospital you can talk to, and you can also access impartial advice from the CAB and cancer charities. If you are caring for someone with cancer, you may be eligible for Carer's Allowance.

Information on benefit entitlement can be found on NHS Choices and Macmillan Cancer Support websites (see help list). There is also a booklet published by Macmillan, entitled *Help With the Cost of Cancer*, which gives you all the information you need to access everything you are entitled to. This is available online or in print and covers Northern Ireland, England, Scotland and Wales.

Helping others

You may find that you are inspired through help that you have received to do something to help others.

Macmillan Cancer Support estimates that two million people are living 'with or beyond cancer', and are campaigning to help everyone in this situation have access to the services and support they require, even years after treatment. If you would like to be involved, visit their website and find out how you can take part. You can comment online, attend a conference or be part of various activities.

Other organisations such as Cancer Research UK, Jo's Trust and local support groups will all offer you opportunities to be involved. You may want to be a 'buddy' for other women, to write articles or books to share your experiences, to campaign to improve services – a whole range of different activities are available.

However, please don't feel that you should do any of these things. Everyone is different and you may feel you want to put the experience behind you and not talk about it to anyone.

Also, you may feel like dipping in and out of involvement with charities or campaigns at various times. Again, this is absolutely fine – just do as much or as little as is right for you.

'You may find that you are inspired by help that you have received to do something to help others.'

Summing Up

This chapter has looked at some of those 'What now?' questions you might be asking yourself, whether you have come through treatment or are about to undergo treatment for cervical cancer.

There is lots of practical advice available from various organisations on coping with the physical and emotional after effects of cancer and the treatment, getting back to work and helping others if you wish.

The help list that follows brings together all those sources of help and suggests some books that may be useful for you.

You may share the experience of many people who say that although they are not glad they have had cancer, some of the outcomes have been positive. For many, the most significant is a renewed appreciation of what is really important to you in your life: family, friends, enjoying nature – all the things that money cannot buy.

You may find, as I do, the 'Serenity poem' a source of support:

'Please grant me the Serenity to accept the things I cannot change,
Courage to change the things I can,
and the Wisdom to know the difference.'
(Anon.)

Help List

Adoption UK
Linden House, 55 The Green, South Bar Street, Banbury, Oxfordshire, OX16 9AB
Tel: 0844 848 7900 (helpline)
helpdesk@adoptionuk.org.uk
www.adoptionuk.org
Provides independent support, information and advice to adoptive parents and foster carers before, during and after adoption.

Cancer Help UK
Tel: 0808 800 4040 (helpline, 9am to 5pm, Monday to Friday)
www.cancerhelp.org.uk

Cancer Research UK
PO Box 123, Lincoln's Inn Fields, London, WC2A 3PX
www.cancerresearchuk.org
The world's leading independent organisation dedicated to cancer research.

Citizen's Advice Bureau
www.citizensadvice.org.uk
With branches all over the country, the CAB offers free advice on finance and legal matters. Visit the website to locate your nearest branch.

European Cervical Cancer Association
121 Rue Jourdan, 1060 Brussels, Belgium
Tel: +32 (0)2 538 2833
info@ecca.info
www.ecca.info
Dedicated to raising awareness of cervical cancer and what can be done to prevent it.

Families Facing Cancer
Tel: 0844 35 77 959
anne@familiesfacingcancer.org
www.familiesfacingcancer.org
Aims to provide emotional and practical support to people affected by cancer.

Health Talk Online

www.healthtalkonline .org

The DIPEx Health Talk website contains interviews, video and audio material of real people talking about their experiences.

Irish Cancer Society

Irish Cancer Society, 43/45 Northumberland Road, Dublin 4, Ireland

Tel: 1 800 200 700 (helpline)

helpline@irishcancer.ie

www.cancer.ie

Charity that aims to achieve world class cancer services in the Republic of Ireland, focusing on prevention, early detection and fighting cancer.

Jo's Trust

16 Lincoln's Inn Fields, London, WC2A 3ED

Tel: 0207 936 7498

robert@jotrust.co.uk

www.jotrust.co.uk

Charity providing easily accessed 'good' information, support and confidential medical advice free of charge 24 hours a day through the website.

Macmillan Cancer Support

89 Albert Embankment, London, SE1 7UQ

Tel: 0808 808 0000 (helpline, 9am to 8pm, Monday to Friday)

www.macmillan.org.uk

Aims to provide a source of support for people affected by cancer, including patients, carers, families and communities.

Macmillan Cancer Support Learn Zone

www.learnzone.macmillan.org.uk

Website dedicated to online learning and development for health professionals, members of the public and Macmillan staff and volunteers regarding cancer.

NHS Cancer Screening Programmes

Fulwood House, Old Fulwood Road, Sheffield, S10 3TH

Tel: 0114 271 1060

info@cancerscreening.nhs.uk

www.cancerscreening.nhs.uk

NHS website providing information on cancer screening programmes in the UK. It also has national statistics and reviews available to download.

NHS Choices

www.nhs.uk

Contains information on all health issues, overviews, expert views, real stories and up-to-date related new stories.

NHS Immunisation Information

Department of Health, Area 511 Wellington House, 133-155 Waterloo Road, SE1 8UG

Tel: 0845 602 3303 (helpline)

www.immunisation.nhs.uk

Provides comprehensive, up-to-date information on vaccines, disease and immunisation in the UK. You can find information relating to the HPV vaccination for cervical cancer here, the helpline number listed is solely for HPV vaccine-related calls.

Teenage Cancer Trust

3rd floor, 93 Newman Street, London, W1T 3EZ

Tel: 020 7612 0370

tct@teenagecancertrust.org

www.teenagecancertrust.org

Teenage Cancer Trust is a charity dedicated to building NHS units specifically for teenagers with cancer.

Teens First for Health

www.childrenfirst.nhs.uk

Provides age-appropriate explanations and advice about a range of health issues. You can contact doctors through the 'dear doc' section on the website.

Teen Info on Cancer

www.click4tic.org.uk

Provided by Macmillan Cancer Support, this website provides honest cancer information written specifically for teenagers.

US National Cancer Institute

www.cancer.gov

Click 'NCI Publications' to access a big selection of booklets that can be viewed online or printed, some are aimed specifically at family, friends and teenagers affected by a loved-one being diagnosed with cancer. Some information may be very specific to the US.

Youth Health Talk

www.youthhealthtalk.org

Part of the DIPEx Health Talk website with interviews, video and audio material of real people talking about their experiences.

Book List

100 Questions and Answers about Cervical Cancer
By Don S Dizon, Michael L Krychman, Paul A DiSilvestro, Jones and Bartlett, USA, 2009.

Adoption and Fostering – A Parent's Guide
By Holly Noseda, Need2Know, Peterborough, 2008.

A Woman's Guide to the Cervical Smear Test
By Anne Szarewski, Random House, Australia, 1994.

Coping Successfully with Your Cervical Smear
By Karen Evennett, Sheldon Press, London, 1996.

Crisis and the Miracle of Love: Mastering Change and Adversity at Any Age
By M Patel and H Waters, Life Foundation Publications, Australia, 1997.

Dare to Blossom: Coaching and Creativity
By Mary Lunnen, Dare to Blossom Books, Cornwall, 2008 (signed copies available from the author).

Dying Well: A Holistic Guide for the Dying and Their Carers
By Richard Reoch, Gaia Books, London, 1997.

Feel the Fear and Do It Anyway
By Susan Jeffers, Vermilion, London, 2007.

Female Cancers, A Complementary Approach
By Jan de Vries, Mainstream Publishing, Edinburgh and London, 2004.

Flying in the Face of Fear
By Mary Lunnen, The Hypatia Trust, New Mill, 1998 (note: the few copies remaining in print are available via the author, price includes a 50p donation to Macmillan Cancer Support).

Happiness Now!
By Robert Holden, Hodder & Stoughton, London, 1998.

Help With the Cost of Cancer
By Macmillan Cancer Support, available online or by phoning 0800 500 800.

Love, Medicine and Miracles
By Bernie S Siegel, Arrow, London, 1998.

Positive Smear
By Susan Quilliam, Charles Letts and Co Ltd, London, 1992.

Preventing Cervical Cancer
By Anne Szarewski, Altman Publishing, St Albans, 2007.

Sexually Transmitted Infections – The Essential Guide
By Nicolette Heaton Harris, Need2Know, Peterborough, 2008.

Shift Happens!
By Robert Holden, Hodder & Stoughton, London, 2000.

Student Cookbook: Healthy Eating – The Essential Guide
By Ester Davies, Need2Know, Peterborough, 2008.

The Pill – An Essential Guide
By Jo Johnson, Need2Know, Peterborough, 2008.

Their Cancer, Your Journey
By Anne Orchard, Rainbow Heart Publishing, Bridport, 2008.

You Can Heal Your Life
By Louise L Hay, Eden Grove Editions, London, 1996.

References

Moore, J, 'Gardasil: a cancer jab I don't regret. Girls of 12-18 will soon be offered a controversial cervical cancer vaccination. Should parents welcome it?', *Sunday Times*, 20 July 2008.

Siegrist, CA, 'Autoimmune diseases after adolescent or adult immunization: What should we expect?', *Canadian Medical Association Journal*, 2007, vol.177, issue 11, pages 1352-4.

Szarewski, A, Adams, M, Briggs, P *et al.*, *HPV vaccination - Moving beyond the current vaccination programme*, MGP Ltd: Berkhamsted, 2009.

Glossary

Adenocarcinoma
A type of cervical cancer that starts in the cervical canal and can, therefore, be more difficult to detect using cervical screening tests.

Benign
A self-contained tumour that is unlikely to grow or spread. Benign tumours can cause problems if they are pressing against surrounding tissues. They can usually be removed by surgery.

Biopsy
A piece of tissue removed from the body to aid diagnosis of a condition or disease.

Brachytherapy
Internal radiotherapy given to cervical cancer patients. The dose can be stronger and with less damage to surrounding tissues and may be more effective in destroying cancer cells.

Cervarix®
One of the two licensed vaccines for use in the HPV vaccination programme.

Cervical intra-epithelial neoplasia (CIN)
CIN refers to abnormal growth and changes in the cells of the cervix, caused by the HPV virus in 99.7% of cases. CIN changes are known as pre-cancerous and can be detected by the cervical screening process. If left, they can develop into cervical cancer.

Cervical screening
Also known as a smear test, cervical screening is where the nurse takes a sample of cells from the cervix to check for any changes.

Cervix
The lower part of the womb (uterus) that forms a passageway and connects the womb to the vagina. It is sometimes called the neck of the womb.

Chemotherapy
The use of drugs to destroy cancer cells. Can be used before surgery or radiotherapy, and in advanced cases can be used alongside radiotherapy.

Clinical oncologist
A medical specialist dealing with the non-surgical forms of cancer treatment.

Cold coagulation
A hot probe used to burn away the abnormal cells in the cervix.

Colposcopy
An examination of the cervix by the doctor using a colposcope, usually after an abnormal cervical screening test result. The doctor will take a biopsy of abnormal cells for further investigation.

Cone biopsy
A larger tissue sample than a biopsy, this may remove the abnormal area if it is small, or be used for diagnosis.

Cryotherapy

A cold probe used to freeze away the abnormal cells in the cervix.

CT scan

CT stands for computerised tomography and is a special kind of x-ray that will result in a two-dimensional image that can be used to plan radiotherapy treatment.

Cytologist

Laboratory staff responsible for checking the smear samples taken during a cervical screening test.

Dyskaryosis

Dyskaryosis literally means 'abnormal nucleus' and refers to the cells taken from the cervical screening test. The cells will be graded as showing mild, moderate or severe dyskaryosis.

Gardasil®

One of the two licensed vaccines for use in the HPV vaccination programme.
Gardasil® is the vaccine currently used by the NHS in the programme.

Genito-urinary medicine (GUM) clinic

Usually based at a hospital, GUM clinics provide sexual health services including testing and treatment for sexually transmitted infections.

Grade

The grade of cancer refers to how quickly it might grow and spread.

Hormone replacement therapy (HRT)

A treatment used to replace hormones that your body is no longer producing itself due to the menopause. If you undergo a hysterectomy or radiotherapy this will create premature and sudden menopause for which HRT can be used to ease the symptoms.

Human papilloma virus (HPV)

A group of over 100 common viruses that can be passed on by skin to skin contact. HPV can cause abnormalities in the cells of the cervix which can lead to cervical cancer. In the UK the NHS are running an HPV vaccination programme that protects against the two most common strains associated with cervical cancer.

Internal radiotherapy

Targeted radiotherapy given through the vagina (also known as brachytherapy) administered to cervical cancer patients. The dose can be stronger and with less damage to surrounding tissues and may be more effective in destroying cancer cells.

Intravenous

Drugs administered to the patient directly into a vein.

Large loop excision of the transformation zone (LLETZ)

A surgical procedure where the area of abnormal cells is removed completely. Also known as loop diathermy.

Late effects

Used to describe side effects that may happen some time after you have finished radiotherapy. Late effects are very rare and it's not possible to explain why some people suffer from them.

Liquid based cytology (LBC)

A new way of preparing cervical screening samples for examination in the laboratory. It reduces the number of inadequate samples from which a result cannot be issued.

Lymph nodes

Lymph nodes are found throughout the body and act as filters or traps for foreign particles. Cancer can spread through the lymph system to other parts of the body, which is why the lymph nodes are used in determining the stage of cancer.

Malignant

A malignant tumour is one that displays uncontrolled growth, invasion of surrounding tissue and can sometimes spread to other areas of the body via the lymph system or blood (also known as metastasis).

Metastasis

The term used when cancer spreads to other parts of the body via the lymph system or blood.

MRI scan

MRI stands for magnetic resonance imaging and involves the patient lying inside a large cylindrical shaped magnet. From this process it is possible to see a picture of almost all of the tissue in the body.

NHS cancer screening programme (NHSCSP)

The national body that is responsible for cancer screening. They closely monitor of all the services concerning cancer screening including the training of nurses and doctors. It also sets the standards for training for taking smears.

Oncology

The branch of medicine that specialises in cancer diagnosis and treatment.

Pre-cancerous

Used to describe symptoms that can, but not always, develop into cancer.

Radical hysterectomy

Also known as a Wertheim's hysterectomy. The womb, the cervix and its surrounding tissue, fallopian tubes, pelvic lymph nodes, the upper vagina and sometimes the ovaries are all removed to minimise the risk of the cancer spreading.

Radiotherapy

The use of radiation to destroy cancer cells. It can be given externally using x-rays, electrons and protons, or internally by drinking a liquid or putting radioactive material in, or close to, the tumour.

Smear test

Also known as a cervical screening test, this is where the nurse takes a sample of cells from the cervix to check for any changes.

Speculum

A tool used to investigate body cavities. For cervical screening it is used to dilate the vagina to examine the cervix and take a sample.

Squamous cell carcinoma

The most common type of cervical cancer. The squamous cells are the flat cells that cover the surface of the cervix.

Squamous epithelium

The layer of cells covering the cervix.

Stage

The stage of cancer describes the size of the cancer and whether it has spread from the original site.

Sexually transmitted infection (STI)

A disease passed on through intimate and sexual contact. Common STIs include chlamydia, gonorrhoea and also HPV strains which can cause cervical cancer.

Trachelectomy

A type of operation for very early stage cervical cancer where the womb and ovaries are not removed so it may still be possible to conceive and carry a baby to term.

Wertheim's hysterectomy

Also known as a radical hysterectomy. The womb, the cervix and its surrounding tissue, fallopian tubes, pelvic lymph nodes, the upper vagina and sometimes the ovaries are all removed to minimise the risk of the cancer spreading.